The Gastroparesis Diet & Cookbook

For Beginners

A Complete Guide to Combating Irritable Bowel Syndrome with Delicious, Healthy Recipes.

Title:

The Gastroparesis Diet & Cookbook

For Beginners

Subtitle

A Complete Guide to Combating Irritable Bowel Syndrome with Delicious, Healthy Recipes.

Copyright © 2023 by (Dr. Rebekah Marvin)

Printed in the United States of America.

ISBN: 9798869620583

TABLE OF CONTENT

CHAPTER 1 1

INTRODUCTION 1

Understanding Gastroparesis 1

Causes And Risk Factors Of Gastroparesis 4

Symptoms Of Gastroparesis 8

Diagnosis And Treatment Options For Gastroparesis 11

The Role Of Diet In Managing Gastrodoresis 15

CHAPTER 2 19

THE GASTROPARESIS DIET 19

Overview Of The Gastroparesis Diet 19

Gastroparesis Diet Foods to Avoid or Limit 24

Approved and Suggestioned Foods for the Gastroplasty Diet...28

Portion Control And Meal Planning For The Gastroparesis Diet...32

Traveling and Eating Out With Gastroparesis...36

Hydration Is Critical In The Gastroparesis Diet...39

CHAPTER 3...42

THE GASTROPARESIS COOKBOOK..42

Gastroparesis Diet Breakfast Recipes....45

Appetizers And Snacks For The Gastroparesis Diet...48

Gastroparesis Diet Main Courses...51

Gastroparesis Diet Desserts and Treats.54

Beverages For The Gastroparesis Diet...57

CHAPTER 4 .... **59**

GASTROPARESIS NUTRITIONAL CONSIDERATIONS **59**

The Role of Macro- and Micronutrients in Gastroparesis Diet 59

Nutrient Deficiencies and Supplementation in Gastroparesis 64

CHAPTER 5 .... **67**

LIFESTYLE MANAGEMENT FOR GASTROPARESIS **67**

Managing the Social and Emotional Consequences of Gastroparesis............ 67

Techniques for Handling Symptoms Associated with Gastroparesis.........**Error! Bookmark not defined.**

CHAPTER 6 .... **70**

GASTROPARESIS AND SPECIAL POPULATIONS............................. **70**

Gastroparesis And Children 70

Gastroparesis And Pregnancy 73

Gastroparesis And Older Adults............ 76

Gastroparesis And Athletes 80

CONCLUSION **83**

APPENDICES **86**

Sample Meal Plans For The Gastroparesis Diet... 86

Common Gastroparesis-Friendly Recipes And Nutritional Information 90

CHAPTER 1

INTRODUCTION

Understanding Gastroparesis

A medical condition known as gastroparesis disrupts the regular movement of food through the stomach. People who have gastroparesis have stomach muscles that do not contract properly or at all, which prevents food from moving through the stomach and into the small intestine promptly. As a consequence of this, food stays in the stomach for a longer period than it ought to, which can result in uncomfortable sensations such as nausea, vomiting, bloating, and abdominal discomfort.

One's risk of developing gastroparesis increases if they have a history of nerve injury, uses certain medications, or suffers from a medical condition such as diabetes or Parkinson's disease. Operation or treatment with radiation might also bring on this condition.

To diagnose gastroparesis, a patient will typically undergo a gastric emptying study. During this procedure, the patient will consume a meal that contains a trace amount of radioactive material and then have their stomach scanned to track the movement of the food as it moves through the stomach. The digestive disorder known as gastroparesis is often treated with a combination of dietary modifications, medication, and, in rare cases, surgery.

In the management of gastroparesis, nutrition plays an essential role. A gastroparesis diet often consists of liquids, pureed or soft foods, and small, frequent meals that are low in fat and fiber. Additionally, the diet may also include foods that are pureed or soft. In addition to this, it is essential to limit your use of alcohol and caffeine.

Causes And Risk Factors Of Gastroparesis

The following is a list of some of the risk factors and reasons that might lead to gastroparesis:

- Gastroparesis is a common complication of diabetes, particularly when blood sugar levels are not well managed.

- It is possible to develop gastroparesis as a consequence of having abdominal surgery that causes damage to the nerves or muscles of the stomach.

- Drugs: Because they slow down the stomach muscle contractions, certain drugs, such as opioids and some antidepressants, might induce gastroparesis in some patients.

- Some neurological conditions can be associated with gastroparesis, including multiple sclerosis and Parkinson's disease.

- The onset of gastroparesis has been related to several different viral diseases, including herpes simplex virus and Epstein-Barr virus, amongst others.

- Gastroparesis can be caused by autoimmune diseases such as scleroderma and lupus, which can damage the muscles and nerves of the digestive tract and lead to impaired digestive function.

- Gastroparesis can be brought on by eating disorders such as anorexia nervosa and bulimia nervosa, both of which can weaken the muscles and nerves of the digestive system.

- Other medical conditions, such as hypothyroidism, gastroesophageal reflux disease (GERD), and some forms of cancer, have also been linked to the development of gastroparesis.

Several variables might increase your likelihood of getting gastroparesis, including being a woman, reaching the age of 40 or older, having a history of diabetes, or having undergone surgery. If you develop symptoms of gastroparesis or have any of these risk factors, you should make an appointment with your primary care physician as soon as possible.

Symptoms Of Gastroparesis

The symptoms of gastroparesis might vary from one individual to the next, however common instances include the following:

- Nausea is one of the most prevalent symptoms of gastroparesis, and it can also manifest itself as an urge to throw up.

- Patients suffering from gastroparesis frequently experience vomiting, particularly after meals.

- Bloating of the abdomen can occur even after a very small amount of food has been consumed, and this can cause the stomach to feel full and bloated.

- Pain or discomfort in the abdomen region is one of the most common signs and symptoms of gastroparesis.

- People who have gastroparesis may find that they feel full more quickly and have less of a desire to eat as a result.

- Weight loss can be an unintended side effect of having gastroparesis, which can cause the condition.

- Heartburn or acid reflux can be the symptoms experienced by a person who has gastroparesis since the condition can cause stomach acid to flow back into the esophagus.

- Blood sugar levels that are not accurate: Diabetics who have gastroparesis may have a difficult time maintaining their blood sugar levels.

- Alterations in bowel movement Gastroparesis can cause either diarrhea or constipation in certain patients.

If you are experiencing any of these symptoms, you should make an appointment with a medical professional to receive an accurate diagnosis and appropriate treatment. Because gastroparesis can be a chronic illness, it is essential to diagnose and treat the condition as early as possible to maintain a high quality of life.

Diagnosis And Treatment Options For Gastroparesis

A diagnosis of gastroparesis often involves looking at a patient's medical history, doing a physical exam, and performing diagnostic testing. These could include the following:

Gastric emptying study: The diagnosis of gastroparesis typically involves this particular test. After the individual eats a meal that contains a minute quantity of radioactive material, their stomach is scanned to monitor the movement of the food through their digestive system.

An upper endoscopy is a diagnostic technique that involves inserting a flexible tube with a camera at the end into the patient's esophagus and stomach to look for any abnormalities or blockages.

Electrogastrography is a method that may determine whether or not there is electrical activity in the muscles of the stomach.

The breath test is used to detect the amount of gas that is produced by bacteria in the stomach.

The digestive disorder known as gastroparesis is often treated with a combination of dietary modifications, medication, and, in rare cases, surgery. The following are many common forms of therapeutic intervention:

Changes in diet: A gastroparesis diet consists of small, frequent meals that are low in fat and fiber, along with liquids and easier-to-digest pureed or soft foods. Drinking plenty of water and avoiding coffee and alcohol are also essential.

Drugs: The symptoms of gastroparesis may be treated with a combination of drugs. These include prokinetic medicines, which aid in stimulating stomach contractions, and anti-nausea drugs.

Botulinum toxin injection: During this procedure, an injection of botulinum toxin is administered into the stomach to relax the muscles and promote gastric emptying.

Enteral feeding: Enteral feeding may be required in really severe cases. To help in the supply of liquid nourishment, a feeding tube is placed into the patient's small intestine.

Surgery: Rarely, a surgical procedure to remove blockages or the use of a gastric electrical stimulator to assist in regulating stomach contractions may be recommended.

See your physician right away if you think you may have gastroparesis so they can properly diagnose and treat you. They can help you create a treatment plan that is suitable for your condition depending on the severity of your symptoms and the underlying cause of your illness.

The Role Of Diet In Managing Gastrodoresis

The management of gastroparesis must always include nutritional support. Because of this illness, it may be difficult for the stomach to empty properly, which can lead to digestive disorders as well as vitamin deficiencies. The following are some of the reasons why proper diet is so important in the therapy of gastroparesis:

Maintaining enough nutrition: People who have gastroparesis may have a difficult time-consuming sufficient amounts of calories and nutrients because the movement of food through the digestive tract is so slow. A meal that is carefully prepared for someone who has gastroparesis can help to ensure that the body obtains the nutrients it needs to function normally.

Symptom management: Some foods have the potential to aggravate the symptoms of gastroparesis, including nausea, vomiting, and abdominal discomfort. A gastroparesis diet may help reduce symptoms by placing an emphasis on meals that are simpler to digest and avoiding foods and drinks that may cause pain.

Preventing problems: Gastroparesis can have serious repercussions for diabetes patients, including decreased nutrient absorption, dehydration, and abnormal blood sugar levels. These problems may be avoided to some extent by maintaining a balanced diet, which supplies the body with the essential nutrients and fluids it needs to function properly.

Supporting general health: A nutritious diet is important for everyone, but it is especially important for those who have gastroparesis. It is helpful to enhance overall health and well-being by consuming a diet that is well-balanced and rich in fruits, vegetables, lean meats, and whole grains.

If you have gastroparesis, you must seek the assistance of a certified dietitian or another healthcare expert to develop an eating routine that is tailored to your specific needs.

They may be able to help you determine which foods are safe to consume and offer guidance on how to maintain a diet that is both healthy and well-balanced. It is possible to manage the symptoms of gastroparesis and avoid complications by following the appropriate food plan.

CHAPTER 2

THE GASTROPARESIS DIET

Overview Of The Gastroparesis Diet

By adhering to a diet known as the gastroparesis diet, people who suffer from gastroparesis may find respite from their symptoms and an improvement in their capacity to empty their stomachs. The diet recommends eating fewer, more frequent meals of a smaller size throughout the day and focuses an emphasis on the consumption of foods that are easier for the body to digest. A general summary of the diet for gastroparesis may be found as follows:

Low-fat foods: By adhering to a diet known as the gastroparesis diet, people who suffer from gastroparesis may find respite from their symptoms and an improvement in their capacity to empty their stomachs. The diet recommends eating fewer, more frequent meals of a smaller size throughout the day and focuses an emphasis on the consumption of foods that are easier for the body to digest. A general summary of the diet for gastroparesis may be found as follows:

Low-fiber foods: Fiber is an important part of a healthy diet, however those with gastroparesis may find it difficult to digest. Choose low-fiber foods like white bread, rice, and pasta in place of high-fiber ones like whole grains, nuts, and seeds if you're trying to lose weight.

Soft or pureed foods: Pureed or liquid meals are easier for the body to digest than solid ones. Another option is to try pureed fruits and vegetables, soups, and protein smoothies.

Smaller, more frequent meals: Smaller meals taken more frequently will aid in better digestion and the relief of discomfort. Strive to eat six to eight smaller meals throughout the day in place of three larger ones.

Liquid foods: It is crucial to drink enough liquids and be well-hydrated throughout the day since they are simpler to digest than solid foods. Soups, broths, and smoothies are more options.

Avoid alcohol and caffeine: Avoiding alcohol and caffeine is crucial since they both have the potential to exacerbate the symptoms of gastroparesis. You ought to try some water or herbal tea instead.

Monitor blood sugar: Blood sugar levels might fluctuate as a result of gastroparesis, thus it's critical to regularly monitor blood sugar levels and adjust diet as needed.

It is essential to work together with a registered dietitian or a healthcare practitioner to develop a nutrition plan that is tailored to your specific needs as well as the kinds of foods and flavors that you enjoy eating. They will be able to aid you in identifying goods that are safe to eat and give guidance on how to maintain a healthy and well-balanced diet while managing the symptoms of gastroparesis. They will also be able to assist you in locating items that are safe to consume.

Gastroparesis Diet Foods to Avoid or Limit

Because they can exacerbate symptoms or slow down the stomach's emptying process, many foods should be limited or avoided entirely while following a diet for gastroparesis. Avoiding or limiting consumption of the following foods is recommended:

1. High-fat foods: Foods that are high in fat can be difficult to digest and may impede the emptying of the stomach. Avoid or restrict your consumption of fried meals, meats high in fat, creamy sauces, and dairy items with a high-fat content.

2. High-fiber foods: Fiber can exacerbate the symptoms of gastroparesis and be challenging to digest. Avoid or consume in moderation whole grains, nuts, seeds, and raw fruits and vegetables.

3. Tough or fibrous meats: Meats that are fibrous or tough, such as steak or pork chops, might be challenging to digest. Opt instead for lean, soft meats such as fish or chicken.

4. Foods that cause gas: Certain meals may result in excess gas in the stomach, exacerbating symptoms. Beans, broccoli, cabbage, onions, and carbonated drinks are to be restricted or stayed away from.

5. Spicy or acidic foods: Foods that are spicy or acidic might increase the symptoms of gastroparesis by irritating the stomach lining. Tomatoes, citrus fruits, spicy food, and products made with tomatoes have to be restricted or avoided.

6. Caffeine and alcohol: Alcohol and caffeine can exacerbate symptoms by slowing down the stomach's emptying process. Avoiding or consuming small amounts of alcohol, coffee, tea, and other caffeinated beverages is advised.

7. Large meals may exacerbate symptoms by overtaxing the digestive system. Rather, strive for smaller, more frequent meals spread out throughout the day.

You must collaborate with a skilled dietitian or healthcare practitioner to determine the foods that trigger your symptoms and to develop a bespoke nutrition plan that addresses your specific needs.

Approved and Suggestioned Foods for the Gastroplasty Diet

Because they facilitate gastric emptying and are simpler to digest, several foods are recommended and safe in the gastroparesis diet. The safe and recommended foods for the gastroparesis diet are as follows:

- Low-fat foods: Healthy gastroparesis diet choices include lean meats like chicken and fish, fruits, and vegetables, as well as low-fat dairy products.

- Low-fiber foods: Foods low in fiber are simpler to digest than those high in fiber, such as cooked vegetables, white bread, rice, and pasta.

- Meals that are soft or pureed are preferable for persons who have gastroparesis because they are simpler to digest. Examples of foods that fall into this category include smoothies, soups, pureed fruits and vegetables, and protein drinks.

- Because liquid meals are easier to digest than solid foods, liquid foods such as broths, soups, and smoothies are appropriate dietary alternatives for people with gastroparesis.

- Meals that are more frequent but smaller Eating meals that are smaller but more frequent throughout the day will help empty the stomach more quickly and ease discomfort.

- Sugary meals have been shown to exacerbate the symptoms of gastroparesis; therefore, it is best to choose low-sugar alternatives, such as fresh fruits, low-sugar yogurt, and sugar-free gelatin.

- foods low in acid Acidic foods can irritate the lining of the stomach, which can make the symptoms of gastroparesis worse. In favor of fruits that are low in acid, such as bananas and melons, you should limit or refrain from eating citrus fruits, tomatoes, and products based on tomatoes.

It is essential to consult with a certified dietitian or a healthcare practitioner to develop a tailored nutrition plan that takes into account your particular requirements and preferences. They will be able to aid you in determining which foods are appropriate for you to eat and provide guidance on how to keep a healthy and well-balanced diet while managing the symptoms of gastroparesis.

Portion Control And Meal Planning For The Gastroparesis Diet

Because they can help reduce symptoms and enhance stomach emptying, meal planning, and quantity management are essential components of the diet for gastroparesis. On a diet for gastroparesis, the following are some ideas for meal planning and controlling portion sizes:

- Make your meals more frequent and smaller: Instead of having two or three large meals per day, try to eat four or six smaller meals each day. This might help to alleviate the discomfort while also promoting the emptying of the stomach.

- Pick foods that are simple for your body to break down: Choose foods that are easy to digest and low in fat, fiber, and sugar such as lean proteins, vegetables that have been cooked, and foods that are soft or pureed.

- Utilize plates of a smaller size: Using plates of a smaller size can help with managing portions and prevent overeating.

- Use spoons and measuring cups to determine how much food you should consume at each meal, and aim for around half to one cup.

- Chew your food completely and slowly if you want to have an easier time digesting it.

- Consuming large quantities of liquids with meals is something that should be avoided because it can slow down the emptying of the stomach. Drink small amounts of liquids frequently throughout the day.

- Keep a food diary to track your symptoms and identify the foods that set off your reaction.

It's crucial to collaborate with a registered dietitian or other healthcare professional to create a customized meal plan and portion management approach that works for you. To assist you in controlling your gastroparesis symptoms and enhance your general nutrition, they can provide you with advice on meal timing, portion sizes, and food selection.

Traveling and Eating Out With Gastroparesis

Eating in restaurants and traveling can be challenging for those who have gastroparesis; nevertheless, it is feasible to keep up a good and balanced diet while on the road with a little bit of planning and preparation ahead of time. When you suffer from gastroparesis, the following are some tips to keep in mind regarding eating out and traveling:

Make a plan: Do your homework on local restaurants and their menus to choose dishes that are suitable for your diet in advance. You may preview the offerings at many restaurants' menus before getting there if they have them posted online.

Keep it simple: Consume meals that are simple to digest and are low in sugar, fat, and fiber content. It is best to steer clear of foods that are fried, hot, and high in fat, as well as raw fruits and vegetables.

Request modifications: You should not feel embarrassed to ask for adjustments to be made to your meal, such as having the vegetables steamed rather than sautéed or asking for the sauce to be served on the side.

Select tiny portions: If you want to take leftovers home, ask for a to-go box or ask for your portion sizes to be reduced.

Sip liquids: During the meal, drinking water or another non-alcoholic beverage that does not include caffeine can facilitate digestion.

When traveling, carry on-the-go foods like nut butter, crackers, and protein bars.

Take into consideration meal replacement shakes or bars: These might be a useful alternative while traveling or dining out.

Speak with your physician: Speak with your doctor about any prescription drugs you might need to take on the road, as well as any extra safety measures you should know about.

Never ignore your body's signals to quit eating if it feels unpleasant or full. Prescriptions, vitamins, and other medical supplies you might need while traveling should also be packed.

Hydration Is Critical In The Gastroparesis Diet

The gastroparesis diet calls for adequate hydration as a fundamental component. People who have gastroparesis have a delayed stomach emptying rate, which can cause them to get dehydrated. This, in turn, can make symptoms such as nausea, constipation, and bloating worse. The following is a list of some of the reasons why drinking sufficient amounts of water is crucial in the diet for gastroparesis:

- Prevents constipation: Constipation is a sign of dehydration and can aggravate the symptoms of gastroparesis. Regular bowel movements and the avoidance of constipation can be achieved by staying hydrated.

- By softening and breaking down food in the stomach and facilitating its easier passage along the digestive system, being hydrated can aid in digestion.

- Boosts vitality: Being dehydrated might make you tired and less energetic. Maintaining your energy levels and improving your general health are two benefits of drinking adequate water.

- Water consumption is a good way to help avoid the bloating and discomfort that come with gastroparesis.

- Prevents issues: Retinal damage is one of the negative effects of severe dehydration, thus it's important to keep hydrated to avoid these health issues.

It's important to drink water throughout the day, even if you don't feel thirsty. Water is the best choice, but low-sugar fruit juices, herbal teas, and sports drinks can also be beneficial. Large volumes of water should not be consumed with meals since this might slow down the emptying of the stomach. Drinking water throughout the day can help you stay hydrated without affecting your digestion. For specific suggestions on hydration and fluid consumption for the management of gastroparesis, speak with a medical professional or qualified dietitian.

CHAPTER 3

THE GASTROPARESIS COOKBOOK

The Gastroparesis Cookbook is a compilation of recipes and meal plans that have been developed specifically for those who are afflicted with the digestive disorder known as gastroparesis. The digestive process can be made more difficult by gastroparesis, which can lead to a variety of uncomfortable symptoms like nausea, vomiting, and bloating. The purpose of this cookbook is to offer recipes for delicious and wholesome meals that are also simple to digest and can be helpful in the treatment and management of gastroparesis symptoms.

This cookbook offers a wide selection of recipes that are low in fat, fiber, and sugar—three components that can make digestion challenging for people who suffer from gastroparesis. Every dish is carefully crafted so that it contains components that are simple to digest and abundant in vital nutrients. In addition, the cookbook provides recommendations for meal planning, guidelines for controlling portion sizes, as well as recommendations for dining out and traveling while suffering from gastroparesis.

Those who suffer from gastroparesis may take advantage of the Gastroparesis Cookbook to prepare a variety of delicious meals that are also good for them, which will help them better control their symptoms and improve their overall health. The cookbook is helpful for anyone who suffers from gastroparesis, as well as their friends and family members who provide care for them.

Gastroparesis Diet Breakfast Recipes

Here are some suggestions for individuals who need to follow a diet due to gastroparesis:

- **Creamy Oatmeal:** Mix one cup of low-fat milk or almond milk with half a cup of rolled oats, then boil until smooth. Add a last touch of honey or maple syrup and a dash of cinnamon.

- **Scrambled Eggs:** Scramble two eggs in a bowl with a touch of butter or olive oil and cook them on a pan that does not stick. A small quantity of low-fat cheese or herbs that have been minced might be added to a dish to impart additional flavor.

- **Smoothies:** Mix until there are no lumps. 1/2 cup of plain Greek yogurt, 1/2 cup of frozen berries, 1/2 cup of low-fat milk or almond milk, and 1/2 cup of plain Greek yogurt.

- **Gluten-free Pancakes:** In a mixing bowl, whisk together 1/2 cup gluten-free pancake mix, 1/2 cup low-fat milk or almond milk, and 1 egg. Cook with a little butter or olive oil on a nonstick skillet. Drizzle with honey or maple syrup and serve.

- **Toast with Nut Butter:** One toasted slice of gluten-free bread spread with a little dollop of peanut butter or almond butter.

Top with berries or sliced banana and serve.

It is important to chew your meal thoroughly and slowly to facilitate digestion. For individualized recommendations about how to best treat gastroparesis with breakfast, speak with a healthcare provider or a registered dietitian.

Appetizers And Snacks For The Gastroparesis Diet

The following is a list of snacks and appetizers that are appropriate for the gastroparesis diet:

Fruit and Yogurt Parfait: 1/2 tablespoon of unsweetened Greek yogurt topped with 1/2 tablespoon of a fruit mixture (such as berries or diced apple). Granola may be sprinkled over top for an extra crunch.

Hummus and Veggies: A snack that is high in protein may be produced by dipping sliced carrots, cucumbers, and bell peppers in a quarter cup of hummus. This creates an appetizing combination that can be eaten on the go.

Rice Cake with Nut Butter: Spread one spoonful of almond or peanut butter over a rice cake to make a snack that will satisfy your appetite. You can also use sunflower seed butter.

Greek Yogurt Dip: Combine one-half cup of plain Greek yogurt, one tablespoon of minced herbs (such as dill or parsley), and a little bit of lemon juice in a blender and mix until smooth. This dip goes well with gluten-free crackers or sliced veggies as a serving accompaniment.

Low-Fat Cheese and Crackers: After spreading a thin layer of low-fat cheese (like goat cheese or cheddar, for example) over gluten-free crackers and then serving the combination, you may make a delectable snack.

Keep in mind that to make digestion easier, snacks should be consumed slowly and in the appropriate amounts. Consult with a healthcare provider or a qualified dietitian if you want tailored guidance on snacks and appetizers for the treatment of gastroparesis.

Gastroparesis Diet Main Courses

The following are some main dish ideas that are permitted on the gastroparesis diet:

1. **Baked Chicken Breast:** A skinless, boneless chicken breast should be seasoned to taste with salt and pepper. Bake for 20 to 25 minutes at 375°F, or until cooked through. Serve with a small portion of cooked rice on the side or with steamed vegetables.

2. **Baked Salmon:** A 4-ounce filet of salmon or cod should be seasoned with salt, pepper, and lemon juice. Bake for 12 to 15 minutes, or until well cooked, at 375°F.

Accompany with roasted vegetables or a small amount of cooked quinoa.

3. **Vegetable Stir-Fry:** Sauté a variety of vegetables in a small quantity of olive or coconut oil (such as bell peppers, zucchini, and broccoli). Garnish with tamari or soy sauce and serve with a small portion of cooked rice or quinoa.

4. To create turkey meatballs, mix ground turkey, minced herbs (such as parsley and thyme), egg, and a small quantity of breadcrumbs. Form into small meatballs and bake at 375°F for 20 to 25 minutes, or until done. Accompany with steamed

vegetables or a small portion of cooked pasta.

5. **Tofu Stir-Fry:** Sauté cubed tofu with a variety of vegetables in a small quantity of coconut oil or olive oil (such as snow peas, carrots, and mushrooms). Garnish with tamari or soy sauce and serve with a small portion of cooked rice or quinoa.

Chewing your food thoroughly and taking your time while eating might improve digestion. Consult a healthcare provider or a competent dietitian for individualized guidance on which main dishes are most suited for the management of gastroparesis.

Gastroparesis Diet Desserts and Treats

Apples in the Oven Begin by coring and slicing one apple, then dusting it with cinnamon. Bake for 15 to 20 minutes at 375 degrees Fahrenheit, or until the vegetables are soft. Serve while still warm, topping each portion with a dollop of vanilla yogurt or whipped cream.

Banana Oat Cookies: One ripe banana, 1/2 cup rolled oats, and a dash of cinnamon should be mashed together. Spoonfuls of the mixture should be placed onto a baking sheet and baked at 350°F for 15 to 20 minutes or until golden brown.

Chia Seed Pudding: In a mixing dish, mix 1/4 cup chia seeds, 1 cup unsweetened almond milk, and a little teaspoon of vanilla extract. Chill the mixture for a minimum of two hours or overnight, or until it becomes thicker. Accompany with freshly cut berries or banana slices.

Frozen Yogurt Bites: Place little dollops of plain Greek yogurt and cut fruit on a baking sheet (such as strawberries or blueberries). Freeze until the mixture is stiff, which should take at least two hours.

Peanut Butter Energy Bites: Mix 1/4 cup rolled oats, 1/2 cup peanut butter, 1/4 cup honey, and a small pinch of vanilla extract.

Roll into little balls and refrigerate for at least an hour before serving.

Keep in mind that you should consume sweets and snacks in moderation and that you should incorporate the amount of sugar and calories that they contain into your overall meal plan. If you need individualized suggestions for gastroparesis desserts and snacks, speak with a healthcare provider or a trained nutritionist.

Beverages For The Gastroparesis Diet

Herbal Tea: Herbal tea is a great substitute for coffee since it naturally contains no caffeine and can soothe upset stomachs. Excellent substitutes include peppermint, ginger, and chamomile teas.

Water: Water consumption is crucial for managing gastroparesis because it keeps the body from becoming dehydrated and constipated. Try to drink eight to ten glasses of water each day.

Low-Fat Milk: High levels of calcium and protein found in low-fat milk are advantageous for those who suffer from gastroparesis. If you are sensitive to lactose, try almond milk or lactose-free milk.

Vegetable Juice: Vegetable juice is simpler to digest than whole vegetables and is rich in vitamins and minerals. Make your veggie juice at home with a blender or juicer.

Smoothies: Smoothies are a great option for those who have gastroparesis since they are nutrient-dense and simple to digest. Blend frozen fruit, yogurt, and a tiny bit of honey to make a tasty and healthy smoothie.

Be sure to ask your treating healthcare provider or a registered dietitian for individualized recommendations on beverages to drink while managing gastroparesis.

CHAPTER 4

GASTROPARESIS NUTRITIONAL CONSIDERATIONS

The Role of Macro- and Micronutrients in Gastroparesis Diet

Because they supply the body with the nutrition it needs to keep its overall health and well-being at a satisfactory level, macronutrients and micronutrients are essential components of the diet for gastroparesis patients.

The body derives a large amount of its energy from macronutrients, which comprise carbohydrates, proteins, and lipids. People who suffer gastroparesis, on the other hand, may have difficulty digesting and absorbing certain macronutrients like fiber and lipids. This can lead to nutritional deficiencies. It is essential, to keep abdominal discomfort at bay, to pick macronutrients that are simple to digest, low in fiber, and low in both fat and calories.

The body receives its source of energy from carbohydrates, which may be found in meals such as fruits, vegetables, cereals, and dairy products. People who suffer from gastroparesis may have a more difficult time digesting carbohydrates that are high in fiber, such as whole grains. Carbohydrates that are low in fiber, including white bread, refined pasta, and cereals that have been cooked should be consumed.

Meals rich in proteins including meat, chicken, fish, lentils, and dairy products are necessary for the growth and repair of tissues. Proteins can be found in a variety of foods. Choose lean proteins like chicken, fish, and low-fat dairy products to alleviate discomfort in the digestive tract by eating these foods.

People who suffer from gastroparesis may have difficulty digesting foods that are high in fat because fats are a source of both energy and essential fatty acids for the body. Consumption of foods that are low in fat, such as lean meats and dairy products with low-fat content, as well as good fats, such as avocado and olive oil, should be done in moderation.

In addition to being necessary for one's general health and well-being, micronutrients such as vitamins and minerals are a good example. People who have gastroparesis run the risk of not getting enough of certain vitamins because they have trouble digesting and absorbing the food they eat. Choose meals that are high in nutrients, such as fruits, vegetables, and lean meats, and think about taking supplements if you feel like you need them.

Overall, it is essential to work with a healthcare practitioner or a registered dietitian to develop a tailored gastroparesis diet plan that fulfills the particular nutritional needs of the patient while also contributing to the treatment of the symptoms of the condition.

Nutrient Deficiencies and Supplementation in Gastroparesis

Patients who have gastroparesis need careful monitoring of their nutritional intake in addition to taking any necessary supplements. Malabsorption of nutrients can be a symptom of gastroparesis, which can lead to nutritional deficiencies.

Gastroparesis is frequently related to dietary deficits of vitamin B12, iron, and vitamin D, as these are some of the most prevalent. Vitamin B12 is almost exclusively present in goods derived from animals and is essential for proper nerve function as well as the production of red blood cells. Iron is essential for the production of hemoglobin, which is responsible for the transportation of oxygen throughout the blood. Vitamin D is necessary for the maintenance of healthy bones as well as the proper operation of the immune system.

To make up for dietary deficiencies, your primary care physician or a skilled dietitian may suggest taking a supplement. To ensure that nutrients are absorbed as well as possible, it may be necessary in some situations to get them by injection or infusion.

People who have gastroparesis need not only take supplements, but they should also have their vitamin levels evaluated. The early diagnosis of deficiencies and the avoidance of their repercussions can be assisted by doing routine blood tests.

It is very necessary to consult with a healthcare provider or a qualified dietitian to develop a customized supplementing and monitoring approach that takes into account unique nutrient demands as well as underlying medical concerns. It is also necessary for one's general health and well-being to consume a diet that is both varied and well-balanced, and which is full of foods that are rich in nutrients.

CHAPTER 5

LIFESTYLE MANAGEMENT FOR GASTROPARESIS

Managing the Social and Emotional Consequences of Gastroparesis

Due to its disruptive effects on daily activities, dietary restrictions, and feelings of loneliness and discontent, living with gastroparesis can have a significant emotional and social impact on people. The following are some coping strategies for the psychological and social effects of gastroparesis:

Getting help: Reaching out to others with gastroparesis or a related condition can be helpful in terms of providing emotional support, sharing experiences, and acquiring coping mechanisms.

Teaching others: Spreading awareness of gastroparesis among friends, family, and coworkers can increase understanding and support while lowering feelings of miscommunication and loneliness.

Enrolling in a support group: Support groups for those with gastroparesis can offer a feeling of camaraderie and encouragement, in addition to the chance to discover novel therapies and coping mechanisms.

People can improve their general well-being, manage stress and worry, and deal with the emotional impacts of gastroparesis by seeing a therapist or counselor.

Engaging in enjoyable and fulfilling pursuits, like hobbies or social events, can improve mood and reduce feelings of loneliness and boredom.

Those with gastroparesis who plan for social events or excursions feel more prepared and in control and experience less anxiety around their dietary choices and symptoms.

CHAPTER 6

GASTROPARESIS AND SPECIAL POPULATIONS

Gastroparesis And Children

Children as well as adults of all ages can suffer from gastroparesis. Many conditions, including nerve damage, medication side effects, and illnesses including diabetes, can result in gastroparesis in children.

Similar symptoms to those experienced by adults, such as nausea, vomiting, stomach discomfort, bloating, and feeling full quickly, can occur in children with gastroparesis. A child's everyday activities, such as eating, playing, and attending school, may be interfered with by these symptoms.

If a kid is diagnosed with gastroparesis, close collaboration between the pediatric gastroenterologist and registered dietitian is essential to the management of the condition. Other treatment options include medication, nutritional and eating behavior modifications, and, in extreme cases, surgery.

It is essential to tailor the approach to the individual needs and preferences of children when it comes to their gastroparesis meals. Children may need smaller, more frequent meals and snacks throughout the day to prevent symptoms. To help them achieve their dietary needs, promote the consumption of nutrient-dense, easily digested meals such as pureed fruits and vegetables.

Children with gastroparesis may experience emotional and social challenges in addition to physical problems. To help them deal with the potential effects that gastroparesis may have on their lives, you must provide them with support and understanding. Counseling and support groups may be beneficial for kids and their families.

Gastroparesis And Pregnancy

It might be challenging to manage gastroparesis during pregnancy. This is because morning sickness, which is common during pregnancy, can be mistaken for gastroparesis symptoms including nausea, vomiting, and bloating. However, gastroparesis can sometimes result in more severe symptoms that could be dangerous for the growing child as well as the mother.

Moreover, pregnancy can change the motility of the gastrointestinal tract and digestion, making gastroparesis symptoms worse. This suggests that to treat their illness, pregnant women with gastroparesis may need to collaborate closely with their healthcare team, which consists of an obstetrician and a gastroenterologist.

The gastroparesis diet may need to be modified during pregnancy to meet the baby's and mother's nutritional demands. To prevent symptoms, this may mean eating more often and consuming nutrient-dense, easily-digested foods. A qualified dietician may offer tailored recommendations based on the stage of the mother's pregnancy and her unique demands.

In addition, pregnant patients with gastroparesis should drink plenty of water and take their prescription drugs as directed by their doctor. In certain situations, hospitalization could be necessary to treat severe symptoms and avoid consequences.

In general, careful treatment and monitoring are necessary throughout pregnancy with gastroparesis to protect the mother's and the unborn child's health and well-being. To get the best outcomes, close coordination with healthcare providers is necessary.

Gastroparesis And Older Adults

A gastroparesis diagnosis can be particularly challenging for elderly individuals, who may already be managing additional medical conditions and dietary issues. To create a customized treatment plan, older adults with gastroparesis must work closely with their healthcare team, which consists of their physician and a licensed dietitian.

Among the potentially helpful therapies for elderly individuals with gastroparesis are:

Frequent monitoring: Diabetes or high blood pressure are two additional health issues that older adults with gastroparesis may have that need to be kept an eye on. Scheduling routine examinations with medical professionals can help guarantee that these ailments are managed properly.

Smaller, more frequent meals: Seniors may not be as hungry or may not be able to handle large portions. Meals should be smaller and more frequent so they can get enough nutrition with the least amount of discomfort.

Soft or pureed foods: Older adults are more likely to experience swallowing and chewing issues. Eating soft or pureed foods that are easy to swallow will help prevent choking and other problems.

Sufficient hydration is important because dehydration can worsen the symptoms of gastroparesis in older people. Maintaining adequate fluid intake throughout the day can help prevent dehydration.

Medication management: The likelihood of drug interactions or adverse effects rises in older adults who may be taking multiple medications. Working in close partnership with a healthcare professional is essential to effectively managing medications and lowering the likelihood of issues.

When older adults with gastroparesis adhere to a prescribed treatment plan and collaborate closely with their healthcare team, they can effectively manage their symptoms and maintain their nutritional status.

Gastroparesis And Athletes

Since gastroparesis impairs an athlete's ability to consume enough food and fluids to satisfy their energy demands, it can be challenging for them to manage. However, with the right care and assistance, athletes with gastroparesis can carry on with their physical activities and sports participation.

Athletes suffering from gastroparesis may find the following strategies helpful:

- collaborating with a trained dietician and a healthcare provider to develop a customized meal plan that addresses their symptoms of gastroparesis and meets their nutritional needs.

- emphasizing nutrient-dense, tolerant foods such as whole grains, lean meats, and fruits and vegetables.

- consuming numerous, smaller meals throughout the day as opposed to bigger, more difficult-to-digest ones.

- drinking well-tolerated liquids, including water or sports drinks, to stay hydrated.

- Trying out various forms of exercise to see which is most comfortable and unlikely to aggravate symptoms of gastroparesis.

- Since stress can exacerbate the symptoms of gastroparesis in some people, stress management is crucial.

- using a network of support to manage the psychological and emotional impacts of gastroparesis, such as a support group or

therapist.

CONCLUSION

To summarize, having gastroparesis can make life challenging at times; nevertheless, with the right mentality and the support of others, it is possible to gain control of the condition and live a life that is full of varied and interesting experiences. The Gastroparesis Diet and Cookbook was written to provide those who are afflicted with the condition of gastroparesis with a wealth of knowledge as well as useful hints that they may implement into their day-to-day life. This material will address subjects such as gaining an awareness of the ailment, its causes and symptoms, the diagnostic process, and the treatment choices available, as well as the necessity of maintaining sufficient diet and hydration. This book offers a wide selection of delectable and healthful recipes that have been modified to meet the needs of individuals who have been diagnosed with gastroparesis. In addition, the book offers guidance on how to modify recipes and offers techniques for meeting nutrient requirements. In addition to this, the book discusses how to live with the emotional and social consequences of gastroparesis, as well as particular concerns for children, pregnant women, elderly people, and athletes. In addition to it, there is an index in the book. If someone with gastroparesis uses this book as a resource, they will be able to take control of their health and well-being, as well as enjoy a diet that is both varied and

satisfying.

APPENDICES

Sample Meal Plans For The Gastroparesis Diet

Meal Plan 1:

- For breakfast, try spinach-topped scrambled eggs and a slice of whole-grain bread.

- Snack: Applesauce with cinnamon.

- For lunch, I had grilled chicken salad with mixed greens, avocado, cucumber, and tomatoes.

- Snack: banana with almond butter.

- Dinner is baked fish over quinoa and roasted vegetables.

Meal Plan 2:

- Breakfast consisted of oatmeal topped with blueberries and a hard-boiled egg.

- Greek yogurt flavored with honey and topped with nuts makes an excellent snack.

- For lunch, I had a sandwich with turkey and cheese, topped with lettuce, tomato, and mustard.

- Oranges cut into slices, accompanied with a handful of trail mix.

- Dinner consisted of turkey meatballs served over zucchini noodles and topped with tomato sauce.

Meal Plan 3:

- Breakfast consisted of a smoothie that included bananas, peanut butter, spinach, and almond milk.

- A snack of baby carrots dipped in hummus with baby carrots.

- For lunch, I had a tuna salad that consisted of mixed greens, cherry tomatoes, and balsamic vinaigrette.

- A snack consisting of rice cake topped with avocado and cherry tomatoes.

- Dinner consisted of baked chicken served with sweet potato and green beans.

Keep in mind that everyone's nutritional needs are different, which is why it is vital to consult with a certified nutritionist to establish a tailored meal plan that responds to both your unique needs as well as your preferences in terms of the foods that you eat.

Common Gastroparesis-Friendly Recipes And Nutritional Information

Certainly, the following is a compilation of recipes that are appropriate for those who suffer from gastroparesis, as well as some nutritional information on a variety of foods and drinks:

Chicken and Vegetable Stir-Fry

Ingredients:

- One tablespoon of olive oil.
- One pound of skinless, boneless chicken breasts finely sliced.
- One cup of carrots, sliced.
- One cup of bell peppers, cut.
- One cup of thinly cut zucchini.

- One tablespoon cornstarch, one tablespoon low-sodium soy sauce.

- Fourteen cups of chicken stock.

- Add salt and pepper to taste.

Directions:

1. Heat the oil in a wok or big pan over high heat.

2. Cook the chicken until it's well done and browned.

3. After taking the chicken out of the pan, set it aside.

4. In the wok, stir-fry the veggies for a few minutes, or until they start to get somewhat soft.

5. In a small bowl, mix soy sauce, cornstarch, and chicken broth.

6. Once the sauce thickens, stir it into the veggies.

7. Add the chicken back to the wok and thoroughly combine.

8. Use salt and pepper to season to taste.

Nutrition information (per serving):

- 295 calories
- 35g of protein
- Fat: 8g
- 18g of carbohydrates
- 4g of fiber
- Salt: 424 mg

Roasted Salmon and Vegetables

Ingredients:

- One-pound fillets of salmon.

- Cut one red bell pepper.

- One slice of zucchini.

- Cut one yellow squash in half.

- One tablespoon of olive oil.

- To taste, add salt and pepper for seasoning.

Directions:

1. One-pound fillets of salmon.

2. Cut one red bell pepper.

3. One slice of zucchini.

4. Cut one yellow squash in half.

5. One tablespoon of olive oil.

6. To taste, add salt and pepper for seasoning.

Nutrition information (per serving):

Calories: 344

Protein: 34g

Fat: 20g

Carbohydrates: 7g

Fiber: 3g

Sodium: 76mg

Banana and Almond Butter Smoothie

Ingredients:

- One ripe banana
- One tablespoon of almond butter

- Half a cup each of basic Greek yogurt and almond milk
- 1/4 tsp vanilla extract 1/4 tsp powdered cinnamon
- Half a cup of cubed ice

Directions:

1. In a blender, combine all the ingredients and process until smooth.
2. If extra ice is needed to get the right consistency, add it.

Nutrition information (per serving):

- Calories: 247
- Protein: 13g
- Fat: 11g

- Carbohydrates: 26g

- Fiber: 4g

- Sodium: 121mg.